BACK PAIN MADE EASY

A Home Guide and Medical Approach for the Relief of Back Pain

Allison E. Clark

Table of contents

INTRODUCTION

Back pain sufferers are acutely aware of how critical it is to find relief. Most people will try to learn as much as they can about their sore back once they are pain-free in an effort to avoid having back problems again.

The upper, middle, and lower backs are just a few examples of how back pain can differ from person to person, type to type, and region to region. It may be a constant, dull ache or an unexpected, dagger-like pain that makes moving almost unbearably painful. If you fall, suffer a sports injury, or lift something too heavy, it can begin quickly. Alternatively, it might get progressively worse over time.

One thing is certain: most people will experience pain at some point in their lives, and it will be memorable. Let's begin by defining back pain and discussing its potential prevalence.

CHAPTER ONE

How common is back pain, and what causes it?

Numerous factors, including those that are structural, musculoskeletal, nerve-based, or indicative of an underlying disorder, can cause back pain. Changes in the structure of the spine can affect the nerves and cause the majority of back pain to be structural or musculoskeletal.

The spine is a complicated network of vertebrae, or interlocking bones and joints. The spinal column runs the full length of our bodies, from the base of the skull to the coccyx, the tailbone at the base of the pelvis. In order for all doctors to know which vertebra they are referring to if there are any back problems that need to be addressed, the numerous vertebrae that make up the spine are labeled in terms of area and each is given a number.

The four locations are as follows, starting with the neck:

- Cervical
- Thoracic
- Sacral and lumbar areas

The lumbar 5, sacral 5, thoracic 12, cervical 7, and thoracic 12 vertebrae are all fused together in the cervical area. In reality, the coccyx is composed of 4 tiny joined bones.

Back pain in the lower back is common. It can affect up to 80% of people at some point in their lives.

Although it is more common in older people and might worsen with age, back pain from an injury can, of course, affect anyone. Gender differences in prevalence exist. Women are more prone to get sciatica, which is pain in the sciatic nerves that run from the back down to the buttocks, lower back discomfort, and a prolapsed or slipped disc.

Furthermore, race has an impact on prevalence. Part of the lower spine slipping out of position in black women is two to three times as common than it is in white women.

What are the primary reasons behind back pain? Let's examine this subject in the following chapter.

CHAPTER TWO

What are the primary reasons behind back pain?

Back discomfort is most frequently brought on by injury. It frequently has to do with lifting up objects in a way that endangers the spine's nerves, surrounding muscles, or both. For instance, when lifting a big object, many people may lean over it with their arms straight and attempt to draw it toward their chest. This puts a strain on the muscles, particularly the muscles in the lower back. Learning good lifting techniques, which we will cover later in this article, can assist avoid back injuries and painful backs.

Anyone can have back discomfort, however, certain factors can make it more likely for you:

<u>Lack of physical fitness:</u>

People who are not fit have back discomfort more frequently. A strong core will also support the back.

<u>weight issue:</u>

Having additional weight, especially around the midsection, can strain and hurt the back. Moreover, it typically indicates a flabby core, and weak, easily injured muscles are a sign of a flabby core.

<u>Heredity:</u>

Certain reasons for back pain may run in families and have a genetic component.

<u>Many health concerns:</u>

Back discomfort can be a symptom of several cancers and kinds of arthritis. Bone spurs, hairline fractures, and other structural changes brought on by osteoporosis, a bone thinning condition, can also result in back pain.

<u>**Cigarette smoking:**</u>

Smokers heal from fractures about twice as slowly as non-smokers. One of the causes can be that the body is not able to circulate enough nutrients to mend bones and sustain healthy back health. Smokers' coughs can cause back pain and even injury as they age because their bones can become so fragile.

<u>**Type of work that you do:**</u>

Your risk of injury increases if your employment frequently requires lifting, pushing, or pulling. Many employers provide back braces for their employees, but for them to be effective, they must be worn properly.

Back discomfort might also occur if you spend all day at a desk and slump forward. Since your lower back bears the majority of the weight and strain when you sit, this region will most often be affected, although it can also affect your neck, shoulders, and middle back.

One of the most typical conditions that leads to discomfort, a low quality of life, and decreased productivity at work is lower back pain. Work, sleep, sex, child care, and other aspects of your life can all be impacted by chronic back pain.

Thankfully, there are a variety of techniques to both prevent and treat back problems. Natural cures, medicines, and in severe situations, surgery are among them. What caused the pain will determine the appropriate remedies.

When there is an injury, it is sometimes extremely clear what caused it. In other situations, the pain is actual, but locating its source and cause may necessitate an eradication procedure.

In an effort to identify the type of pain and its location and determine the cause and the best course of treatment, doctors categorize the pain. The next chapter will examine several types of back discomfort.

CHAPTER THREE

Forms of Back Pain

Upper, middle, and lower back pain will be categorized. They'll also say whether the discomfort is coming from the left or the right. This may offer a hint as to which kind of the several causes of back pain is perhaps causing the patient's problem.

Back pain can have a variety of reasons, broadly categorized as:
- Structure
- Achy muscles
- a painful nerve
- inflammation brought on by conditions like arthritis

There are three standard categories for back pain:

1. An axial ache:

The most common cause of this, also known as mechanical pain, is a strained or sprained muscle. It could be blunt or pointed.

2. Referred Pain:

Referred pain travels from one place to another. It is dull and achy in nature and linked to changes in the spine brought on by aging.

3. Radiating pain

The arm or leg may become numb or weak due to this nerve discomfort, which frequently radiates outward along the route of the afflicted nerve. It is described as intense pain. There are a variety of causes for this pain, including:

• Inflammation,

• Damage to a spinal nerve root and • Nerve compression.

The most typical type of radiating pain is sciatica (SIGH-at-tic-ah). Sciatica is primarily brought on by:

• **a herniated disc**, which is a ruptured disc that may be pressing on a nerve.
• **Degenerative disc disease**, which is a spinal condition brought on by age
• **spinal stenosis**, which is the spine's narrowing
• **Spondylolisthesis**, in which one of the vertebrae slides forward onto the bone below it, compressing or pinching the nerve

Back discomfort that radiates to the hip and thigh is known as sciatica. In some circumstances, it might even extend all the way to the big toe. Which vertebra is being affected will determine this. For instance, if the Lumbar 3 (L3) disc is causing it, discomfort may radiate to the thigh and/or buttocks. The pain may extend all the way to the big toe if the L% is compromised. Thus, it will be crucial to use diagnostic imaging to ascertain the state of the spine and the location of the discs.

Sciatica symptoms that point to an emergency should be treated right away. Among them are, but not restricted to:

• advancing neurological symptoms include numbness or weakness in the legs
• malfunction of the bladder or bowel, or the inability to control pee or feces.

These symptoms can indicate cauda equina syndrome, an uncommon illness characterized by intense pressure and swelling of the nerves near the spinal cord's tip.

Sciatic pain can also be brought on by infection or spinal tumors, so it's crucial to seek treatment rather than just accepting your discomfort as a normal part of getting older.

Lordosis

The abnormal inward curve of the spine known as lordosis is another factor in lower back discomfort. It is frequently called a "sway back." Age or bad posture may be the culprit. Physical therapy is typically utilized as a form of treatment, but in more severe circumstances, surgery, casts, and/or bracing may be needed to restore the spine's natural curve and relieve any pain.

Although the lower back is the most frequently affected area, the upper back can also hurt for musculoskeletal causes and is frequently associated with shoulder pain. Although it is less mobile and flexible than the lower part of the spine, this region of the spine is nevertheless susceptible to injury in accidents.

Dowagers' hump

Kyphosis, also known as the "dowager's hump," is an unnatural outward curvature of the thoracic vertebrae in the upper back. Consider it to be the inverse of lordosis. It frequently happens as a result of osteoporosis, or bone thinning. A hump-like appearance results from the spine's bending. The name comes from the fact that older women, who are much more prone to osteoporosis, frequently exhibit it. The hump can often be removed because osteoporosis is preventable.

Any part of the back may be affected by scoliosis (pronounced SKOL-ee-OH-siss). It results in an abnormal side-to-side curvature of the spine. Scoliosis patients' spines can curve to the point where they start to resemble the letters C or S. This can happen on either side of the spine.

Approximately twice as many women as men experience scoliosis. It can begin at any age, but people over 10 are typically most susceptible. It is inherited and runs in families.

Different curve severity and location factors can result in a variety of symptoms. Surgery is one form of treatment, as well as spinal manipulation and bracing.

Middle and upper back pain
The ribs and each of the 12 thoracic vertebrae that make up your upper and middle back are interconnected on a very fine scale. Therefore, a variety of factors, such as the following, can contribute to middle and upper back pain:

Back pain in the upper and middle back may result from:

muscular overuse, injury to the muscles, ligaments, and discs supporting the spine due to a muscle strain, improper posture, spinal nerves under pressure, perhaps as a result of a herniated disc, one of the vertebrae has fractured, Osteoarthritis, or degeneration of the spine,

Because the discs that cushion the spine's small facet joints begin to degenerate, the spine shrinks and compresses with age. The key to keeping your discs healthy is to take care of your cartilage. A, B6, C, and E vitamins are all crucial. Likewise, copper and zinc are minerals. Along with getting enough hydration, high-quality protein is also necessary.

Your spine can stay healthy if you consume bone broth and leafy greens like spinach and kale. Once you know how, it's simple to make bone broth, which is a delicious way to get the most nutrition out of any animal bones you may have at home, like the carcass from a rotisserie chicken or a leg of lamb.

The connective tissue of a muscle or group of muscles is impacted by myofascial pain, which can also result in back pain in these regions.

CHAPTER FOUR

Which doctors specialize in treating back pain, and when should you see one?

If you encounter:

• Lack of bladder and bodily function control; shooting or stabbing sensations in the back; back muscle spasms; discomfort radiating down one or both legs; restricted flexibility or range of motion in the back;

See a doctor right now.

Additionally, get medical help if the pain persists for longer than two weeks.

Go to the emergency room for a thorough examination if a fall or other injury is the cause. Any medical condition that is detected early usually has the best prognosis.

Back pain specialists in medicine.

Patients with spinal conditions are treated by a variety of different medical professionals. Each has a tad bit of a different specialty or focus. The doctor(s) you visit will be determined by the pain's symptoms and causes.

Typically, visiting your primary care physician (PCP) or a medical professional at your neighborhood emergency room or emergency department will be your first step. After evaluating your condition, they will suggest a course of treatment and may also refer you to one or more other back doctors. These could incorporate:

- Chiropractors to move soft tissues and the spine,

- A doctor of osteopathic medicine (DO) focuses on the body's musculoskeletal system and its overall health.
- A surgeon and other spinal experts.
- Physical or occupational therapist to aid in the healing process following an injury.
- A professional in pain management.

Other experts who can aid in the relief of back pain include:

Nerve problems are handled by **neurologists**.

Rheumatologists treat conditions related to arthritis and other arthritic joints.

Clinicians of complementary and alternative medicine

The objective is to make you as pain-free as possible. In severe cases, this may entail taking medication or having surgery, but more frequently, it may entail making lifestyle changes and attending spine school, which teaches people how to better take care of their spines. It might also include mind-body medicine, particularly for how pain is perceived and how to get rid of it naturally.

On your path to a pain-free back and a healthy spine and body, a variety of CAM practitioners can help. CAM, or complementary and alternative medicine, has a variety of advantages. As their name implies, they can be used in conjunction with other treatments, or in addition to them, with little to no risk of negative side effects. Most insurance companies have CAM provisions in their policies, and CAM is becoming more and more accepted as a way to get treatment for a variety of medical conditions. Later on in this guide, we'll talk about CAM for a sore back.

Of course, there is also you. The best way to maintain a healthy back and, if at all possible, avoid injuries is to take care of your own body and back.

If you do have a sore back, taking preventative measures and adhering to each practitioner's recommended course of treatment—which may include exercises—can speed up your recovery and, ideally, prevent permanent damage to your back.

Let's examine CAM and other natural remedies for a sore back in the following chapter.

CHAPTER FIVE

Natural remedies for easing back pain

Back pain can be treated naturally in a number of ways. It's good to know that many of them are free or reasonably priced. They should, in general, be useful for the upper, middle, and lower back, though their effectiveness will depend on where and what is causing the discomfort.

<u>Self-care:</u>

- not sitting for long periods of time, which puts a lot of pressure on the spine;
- gentle, easy stretching;
- gently working out your core muscles—work on your abs;

- yoga for stretching, increasing flexibility, and improving core strength—try plank pose;
- cold therapy—ice packs or an Icy-hot patch can help;
- heat therapy—a warm bath or shower, heating pad, or electric blanket.
- Aim for 8 hours of good quality sleep each night. Sleep on a bed that provides adequate support for your back. The mattress shouldn't be too soft. Search for orthopedic mattresses; use the proper pillows to prevent neck pain; and use certain medical pillows to support the neck. When sitting, a wedge-shaped pillow placed beneath your backside will support your hips and spine.
- Making sure you are walking correctly in good shoes, avoiding high heels, and taking care of your feet.
- Getting a specially-shaped wedge pillow to put between your thighs to help with sciatic pain when you sleep

at night. Corns, calluses, and other foot conditions can result in discomfort and odd walking patterns.

- Regular exercise, choosing low impact workouts like walking, swimming, cycling, yoga, tai chi, light weights, and resistance bands.
- Correctly lifting heavy objects, including children and pets.
- If you're like most people, spending hours at a desk each day can damage your back if you're not careful. (I'll talk more about this later)

<u>Complementary and Alternative Medicine (CAM):</u>

There are numerous CAM practices that have been shown to reduce pain. Here are some recommendations:

1. You can focus your attention during meditation to relieve stress and discomfort.

2. Talk therapy, also known as cognitive behavioral therapy (CBT),CBT can aid with pain and stress relief. Moreover, it can reduce muscle tension.

3. **controlled relaxation**: For less tension, you will learn to tighten and then release your muscles. Back discomfort is largely caused by tension and stiffness.

4. **Chinese herbal medicine** (TCM): TCM incorporates acupuncture and acupressure for back pain. Both energize the body's "meridians," or energy centers, to support wellness and recovery. Little, delicate needles are used in acupuncture. Hands are used for acupressure.

5. Massage therapy, either by a friend or family member or by a trained

massage therapist, can reduce pain and tension in the muscles.

6. **Aromatherapy:** Essential oils are plant extracts that are used in aromatherapy for health and healing. Essential oils can be applied topically during a therapeutic massage, added to bathwater, or inhaled. Back pain can be relieved by using essential oils that encourage calm and relaxation, such as lavender, rose, and pine.

7. **Physical exercise:** You can receive gentle manipulation and an exercise regimen from a sports clinic or physiotherapist to relieve your back pain and prevent further injury.

8. **Spine traction and decompression:** The spine can be stretched in a variety of ways to release pressure from compressed discs and nerves.

9. pain management professional: A pain management specialist can provide you with a variety of options, such as medication or herbal treatments, to help your back feel better.

It will be time to look at the medications available for lower back pain relief if you try all of these self-care and complementary and alternative medicine (CAM) methods and you are still experiencing back pain.

CHAPTER SIX

Medications to relieve back discomfort

There are numerous potent painkillers available, both over-the-counter and on prescription. Their potency, outcomes, and potential adverse effects differ. Your decision will partly be influenced by how painful your back is. The majority of doctors will ask you to rate your level of discomfort on a scale of 0 to 10, with 0 being no pain and 10 representing significant agony. S/he will offer a variety of recommendations for the treatment(s) that will be most successful based on your pain level and the suspected causes of your back pain.

They might advise:

- painkillers,

- Muscle relaxants,
- drugs that influence the brain's pain centers.

The painkillers can also be found in a variety of forms, such as pills, injections, and pain patches.

Always talk to your doctor about any potential side effects before taking any painkillers. To prevent unintentional overdose, take the medication exactly as directed and according to the recommended schedule.

The most popular back pain medications are:

Acetaminophen (Tylenol)

Although Tylenol is efficient, the possibility of an overdose, which can seriously harm the liver, makes it potentially hazardous. Take exactly as directed, and be sure you haven't taken any other medications—such as cold and flu remedies—that can contain Tylenol and result in an unintentional overdose.

Non-steroidal anti-inflammatory (NSAIDS).

Several over-the-counter drugs, including ibuprofen and naproxen, aid in reducing inflammation, one of the causes of pain. You'll know what inflammation can do to your back and to your entire body if you've ever whacked your thumb with a hammer.

Unprescribed creams

Pain relief can be obtained by applying creams or other topical medications directly to the injured region. If you have a sensitivity to aspirin, be sure to carefully read the labels. Others contain capsaicin, a compound derived from chilies that can burn skin that is already sensitive. Arnica is a natural remedy for pain and bruising that doesn't have a distinct fragrance.

non prescription painkiller patches

The selection of pain treatment patches at the pharmacy is getting larger. Salonpas and Icy Hot are two well-known brands. You should watch out for allergies, irritability, and itching at the patch's site as they each contain distinct active components, such as aspirin and capsaicin.

Muscles relaxants

This group of drugs help ease the soreness and muscular spasms that frequently accompany back pain. Drugs that are frequently administered include Valium and Soma (carisoprodol) (diazepam). However, because both of them have the potential to become habits, they should only be used temporarily.

Painkillers based on opioids

Opiates are effective painkillers that can be used to treat back pain that is acute and has not responded to other medical procedures or medications. Among the drugs in this class are:

Fentanyl, Hydrocodone, Oxycodone, and Codeine.

Because they have a high potential for addiction, they should only be used briefly and in the smallest amount possible.

Antidepressants

Elavil (amitriptyline) and Cymbalta (duloxetine), two antidepressants, can treat depression and, in some situations, chronic pain. They influence the brain's pain receptor areas and improve mood.

Additional drugs that are occasionally prescribed for low back pain include:

Injections with anesthetic

Through the use of anesthetics, a variety of injections are utilized to treat lower back pain. Injections into trigger points aim to target the precise location of the discomfort.

Facet joints, which are the points where two vertebrae of the spine meet, are injected with anesthesia.

Shots of steroids

Inflammation can be reduced by steroids. To relieve pain in and around the spinal column, epidural injections are administered into the spinal canal. Steroids, like any drugs, can have unwanted effects, some of which can be serious, such as glaucoma and high blood pressure.

Anticonvulsants

In some cases, these are employed to relieve low back discomfort. The most widely used are Tegretol (carbamazepine), Neurontin (gabapentin), Dilantin (phenytoin), and Lyrica (pregabalin). Approximately 3 out of 10 persons use gabapentin and see some relief.

Botox

Botox is frequently used for cosmetic purposes to relax and smooth facial muscles and wrinkles. Chronic low back pain is one of the many other health conditions for which it is being utilized. It can ease muscle tension and lessen spasms.

Before starting treatment, go over every potential adverse effect with your doctor. To try to reduce the chance of side effects, let them know what prescription medications, vitamins, and herbal supplements you are using.

It might be time to think about surgery if you have tried a variety of drugs but are still dealing with persistent pain. Next, let's examine your possibilities.

CHAPTER SEVEN

Surgical back pain treatments

It might be time to think about your surgical alternatives if self-care, natural remedies, over-the-counter, and prescription pharmaceuticals are still unable to provide you with pain relief, your back pain has continued for longer than three months, or it has a clear structural cause.

In addition to the standard risks of anesthesia-related problems and surgical site infections, each style of surgery has a number of advantages. Before deciding to have the surgery, make sure you are well informed about the procedure, the reasons behind it, the alternatives, and the likely results.

Sprain Fusion

The most popular operation for back discomfort is spinal fusion. In order to limit motion between the vertebrae of the spine and prevent damage to the nerves and discs, a surgeon may connect one or more vertebrae together. You can have restricted flexibility and range of motion in the vertebra where the fusion has occurred. The discs can occasionally not merge completely. There is a danger of infection, and smokers are more likely to contract an infection and heal more slowly.

Laminectomy.

Spurs are lumps, bumps, and protrusions that can develop on the spine as it ages. They may put pressure on discs, ligaments, or nerves. Your surgeon will remove pieces of the bone and/or bony spurs during a laminectomy to relieve any pressure that may be causing your back discomfort or leg paralysis. A laminectomy's biggest risk is that it can weaken the spine even more. You might require spinal fusion surgery if this occurs. Depending on what the surgeon discovers once he enters, both surgeries may occasionally be carried out at the same time.

Foraminotomy

Your surgeon will perform this procedure to expand the opening where the nerve roots leave the spine by removing part of the bone from the sides of the vertebrae. By doing this, spinal stenosis pressure and discomfort can be relieved. Moreover, this has the potential to weaken the spine, in which case spinal fusion surgery would also be required.

Discectomy.

The discs in your back act as little cushions to keep your vertebrae from grating against one another. The discs in your spine act as shock absorbers to prevent vertebral fracture. They get thinner as they age, but they can also bulge or move around. A spinal nerve may be pressed against as a result. A discectomy involves removing all or a portion of the disc. Depending on your symptoms, this treatment may also be combined with a spinal fusion, laminectomy, or foraminotomy. A prosthetic disc may occasionally be implanted to provide support and widen the space between the vertebrae.

<u>Replacement of the disc</u>

A damaged disc is removed during disc replacement surgery, and an artificial disc is then inserted. Because it still permits a significant amount of motion and flexibility, it is starting to gain popularity as a substitute for spinal fusion. Moreover, recuperation times are typically shorter. The biggest risks are infection, the new disc being rejected, or the disc shifting out of position once more.

<u>Implant interlaminar</u>

Implanting a device at the same time as a laminectomy is another alternative to spinal fusion. In order to release pressure from any potential pinched nerves, the U-shaped device is inserted between two vertebrae. It can aid in reducing the signs and symptoms of spinal stenosis, a narrowing of the spine that may pinched nerves. Although a person with an implant may not be able to bend backwards in that area, it will help maintain mobility and stability in the spine in comparison to fusion.

Back surgery risks

Having back surgery comes with a number of hazards, in addition to the possibility of not experiencing the pain alleviation anticipated. They consist of:

• Bleeding
• Infection
• Blood clots, including as in the legs or lungs, especially if you are bedridden for a prolonged period of time • Heart attack • Stroke • Disc rupture despite the operation

Another danger is spinal nerve injury, which can cause a variety of symptoms, such as:

Inability to regulate one's bowels or bladder, sexual dysfunction, paralysis, weakness, and chronic discomfort (incontinence)

Maintain regular communication with your doctor to ensure the best outcome. To build and maintain a healthy back, use CAM and pharmaceuticals as necessary.

Using the proper lifting technique for large objects is one of the best methods to keep your back in good shape. Let's examine this subject in the following chapter.

CHAPTER EIGHT

How to properly carry objects that are heavy

The greatest approach to prevent damaging your back's structure or harming its muscles is to lift big objects correctly.

1 - Stand

Your dominant foot, such as your right, should be slightly in front of the other while you stand close to the object with your feet shoulder distance apart.

2 - Squat

Squat down next to the item, bending just at the hips and knees while maintaining a straight spine. One knee may be on the floor, but the other must maintain a 90-degree angle.

3 - Remain erect

The shoulders should be back, the back straight, and not slumped. The head need to be up and directed directly ahead.

4 - Align your legs.

Straighten your hips and knees to ensure that your muscles, not your back muscles, are lifting the weight off the ground.

5 - No swaying

Keep your back straight while you use your legs to lift yourself off the ground. Avoid twisting from side to side as this could harm your lower back muscles or entrap a nerve.

6 - Keep it tight and stable.

As closely as you can to your body, hold the load. Avoid stooping over it. Lift it up until it is roughly at your hip and waist level. NEVER attempt to lift it above your shoulders.

7 - Taking baby steps.

With your burden, move ahead gradually. Avoid attempting to walk normally because it may jar your hips and back and potentially cause you to lose your grasp and drop the object.

8 - Swap directions with care.

While changing directions while carrying a large object, you should lead with your hips rather than your feet or knees.

9 - Remain centered

While you move, keep your shoulders and hips in alignment.

10 - Gently establish

Don't extend your arms if you need to place your burden on a table or shelf. Slide the weight on top of the resting area after approaching it as closely as you can. Reverse the lifting procedure if you plan to place it on the floor once more. until the object is once more securely on the ground, squatting just with the knees and hips while maintaining a straight, untwisted back.

You'll be far less likely to pick up large boxes incorrectly because you are not thinking when the time comes if you repeatedly practice this sequence of movements with a tiny, light-weight box until it seems comfortable and natural.

Everyone who has ever had back pain will understand how awful it can be, how much it can impair your quality of life, and how much it can keep you from performing your most basic daily tasks. According to estimates, back discomfort costs the US $240 BILLION annually, not including lost productivity at work and at home.

Back discomfort can have a detrimental effect on every aspect of your life, including your relationships with your partner, kids, and other family members as well as your personal finances, employment opportunities, and job satisfaction. Back pain might interfere with your ability to sleep, feel happy, and enjoy life. Fortunately, if you take care of your back so that it can take care of you, a lot of this may be avoided.

Many people have to deal with back discomfort, but it doesn't have to make your life miserable. You can find a variety of efficient methods to help repair and strengthen your back for better back health by practicing proper self-care, using natural therapies over time, and consulting your doctor.

My best to your back!

Resources

The back pain health center
http://www.webmd.com/back-pain/default.ht
m

Upper and middle back pain
http://www.webmd.com/back-pain/tc/upper-a
nd-middle-back-pain-overview

Lower back pain relief at home
http://www.webmd.com/back-pain/guide/ho
me-relief-for-low-back-pain

Understanding back pain
http://www.webmd.com/back-pain/guide/und
erstanding-back-pain-basics

What you need to know about sciatica
http://www.spine-health.com/conditions/sciat
ica/what-you-need-know-about-sciatica

Spine School

http://www.healthcentral.com/chronic-pain/c/
23153/58933/spine-school/

Spine Specialists
http://www.spine-health.com/treatment/spine
-specialists

Review of Complementary and Alternative
Therapies for Back Pain
http://www.ncbi.nlm.nih.gov/pmc/articles/PM
C3236015/

Complementary and alternative therapies
for back pain II.
http://www.ncbi.nlm.nih.gov/pubmed/231265
34

Nonpharmacologic therapies for acute and
chronic low back pain: a review of the
evidence for an American Pain
Society/American College of Physicians
clinical practice guideline.
http://www.ncbi.nlm.nih.gov/pubmed/179092
10